300 Questions and Answers in Diagnostic Aids for Veterinary Nurses

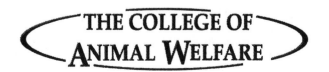

THE COLLEGE OF
ANIMAL WELFARE

Senior commissioning editor: Mary Seager
Development editor: Caroline Savage
Production controller: Anthony Read
Desk editor: Angela Davies
Cover designer: Helen Brockway

300 Questions and Answers in Diagnostic Aids for Veterinary Nurses

The College of Animal Welfare

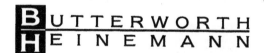

OXFORD AUCKLAND BOSTON
JOHANNESBURG MELBOURNE NEW DELHI

Butterworth-Heinemann
Linacre House, Jordan Hill, Oxford OX2 8DP
225 Wildwood Avenue, Woburn, MA 01801-2041
A division of Reed Educational and Professional Publishing Ltd

Ⓡ A member of the Reed Elsevier plc group

First published 2001

British Library Cataloguing in Publication Data
300 questions and answers in diagnostic aids for veterinary nurses
  1. Veterinary nursing – Examinations, questions, etc.
  2. Veterinary medicine – Diagnosis – Examinations, questions, etc.
  I. College of Animal Welfare II. Three hundred questions and
answers in diagnostic aids for veterinary nurses
636′.089′073′076

ISBN 0 7506 4795 5

Typeset by Keyword Typesetting Services, Wallington
Printed and bound by Antony Rowe Ltd, Eastbourne

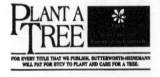

FOR EVERY TITLE THAT WE PUBLISH, BUTTERWORTH-HEINEMANN
WILL PAY FOR BTCV TO PLANT AND CARE FOR A TREE.

Contents

Acknowledgements

The College is most grateful for the help of the following colleagues in the preparation of this book:

C. Allan
B. Cooper
W. Fulcher
D. Gould
A. Jeffery
H. Orpet
A. Thomas

Introduction

How the book is organized

This book of Diagnostic Aids questions has been produced in response to further requests for more multiple choice questions. It contains 300 questions covering diagnostic aids. After the questions is a list of correct answers.

How to use the book

Do your revision first, then select a range of question numbers at random. Do this without looking at the questions in advance. You should be able to complete and finish one multiple choice question per minute, allowing time for a thorough read of the question and the options before selecting the correct answer.

Questions

1) *Toxoplasmosis in people can be prevented by any ONE of the following methods with the EXCEPTION of:*
   a) emptying the cat's litterbox weekly
   b) covering the children's sandbox
   c) washing hands thoroughly before eating
   d) cooking all meats thoroughly before eating

2) *Concerning viruses, which statement is LEAST accurate?*
   a) Viruses do not grow on artificial media and require living cells to grow
   b) Viruses do not have cellular organelles for metabolism
   c) Viruses contain both DNA and RNA
   d) Viruses do not contain ribosomes

3) *The incubation period of a disease is:*

   a) at the height of the illness
   b) before the animal shows clinical signs
   c) once the animal has recovered
   d) once the animal has shown clinical signs

4) *Which ONE of the following diseases is zoonotic:*

   a) canine parvovirus
   b) canine distemper
   c) canine hepatitis
   d) leptospirosis

5) *An example of a pathogenic yeast is:*

   a) Aspergillus sp
   b) Trichophyton
   c) Candida
   d) Microsporum canis

6) *What size (roughly) are viruses?*

   a) Nanometres, nm (1×10^9m)
   b) Micrometres, μm (1×10^6m)
   c) Picometres, pm (1×10^{12}m)
   d) Millimetres, mm (1×10^3m)

7) *Rubarth's disease is:*

   a) an early term for fits
   b) an inherited blood clotting disorder
   c) canine distemper
   d) infectious canine hepatitis

8) *Cigar-shaped mites in a skin scraping from a dog are most likely of the genus:*

   a) Sarcoptes
   b) Notoedres
   c) Otodectes
   d) Demodex

9) *In dogs, a Wood's lamp can sometimes be used to diagnose infection with:*

   a) Microsporum canis
   b) Trichophyton mentagrophytes
   c) Sarcoptes scabiei
   d) Trichophyton verrucosum

10) *Mites in the ear of a dog are typically:*

   a) Sarcoptes scabiei
   b) Notoedres cati
   c) Otodectes cyanotis
   d) Trixacarus caviae

11) *Small, dandruff-like flakes on the hair of a dog appear to move. Examination of the apparent dandruff reveals it to be comprised of mites. This 'walking dandruff' is associated with infestation by:*

   a) Sarcoptes scabiei
   b) Otodectes cyanotis
   c) Cheyletiella yasguri
   d) Trixacarus caviae

12) *Dogs typically acquire Demodex infestations from:*

   a) the bitch as pups while nursing
   b) wild rodents
   c) birds
   d) contact with infested people

13) *How do children get toxocariasis?*

   a) By ingestion of raw meat
   b) By direct contact with dogs infected with roundworms
   c) By ingestion of roundworm eggs in dog faeces
   d) By inhaling aerosol from infected animals

14) *Visceral larval migrans in people is caused by:*

   a) Toxoplasma
   b) Toxocara
   c) Ancylostoma
   d) Echinococcus

15) *An example of an ectoparasite found in the guinea pig is:*

   a) Cheyletiella yasguri
   b) Otodectes cyanotis
   c) Sarcoptes scabiei
   d) Trixacarus caviae

16) *Which ONE of the following is described as being host specific?*

   a) Flea (Ctenocephalides)
   b) Harvest mite (Neotrombicula)
   c) Louse (Trichodectes)
   d) Tick (Ixodes)

17) *Which ONE of the following endoparasites is responsible for hydatidosis?*

   a) Dipylidium caninum
   b) Echinococcus granulosus
   c) Toxocara canis
   d) Trichuris vulpis

18) *The mite Demodex canis appears under the microscope as:*

   a) cigar-shaped with long legs
   b) cigar-shaped with short legs
   c) round with short legs
   d) round with long legs

19) *Bacteria that are spherical in shape and arranged in groups are known as:*

    a) bacilli
    b) spirochaetes
    c) staphylococci
    d) streptococci

20) *Which ONE of the following bottles should be used for storing large volumes of a solution?*

    a) Reagent bottle
    b) Winchester bottle
    c) Dropping bottle
    d) McCartney bottle

21) *The cause of feline infectious anaemia is:*

    a) feline leukaemia virus
    b) coronavirus
    c) parvovirus
    d) Haemobartonella felis

22) *Which ONE of the following is a burrowing mite?*

    a) Cheyletiella Spp
    b) Octodectes cyanotis
    c) Demodex canis
    d) Trichodectes canis

23) *Which ONE of the following is a sucking louse?*

   a) Felicola subrostratus
   b) Sarcoptes scabiei
   c) Linognathus setosus
   d) Ctenocephalides felis

24) *In which of the following bodily fluids might you find leptospira organisms, in an infected animal?*

   a) Gut secretions and faeces
   b) Blood
   c) Urine
   d) Both blood and urine

25) *Chlamydia infection in a cat can be diagnosed using which diagnostic technique?*

   a) Cite test
   b) Microscopy of conjunctival swab
   c) Haematology
   d) Microscopic examination of lacrimal fluid

26) *What is a fomite?*

a) Another host that carries an organism and in which the organism passes part of its life cycle

b) An inanimate object, contaminated by an infected animal, that comes into contact with a non-infected animal

c) Another host that carries the organism and can shed it at any time

d) Another host that carries the organism and has to be eaten to pass on the infection

27) *Which part of the urine stream is used in bacteriological investigations?*

a) the first part of the sample

b) the middle part of the sample

c) the last part of the sample

d) any of the above

28) *How soon after collection should urine be examined, if no preservatives are used?*

a) Within 24 hours

b) Within 6 hours

c) Within 2 hours

d) Within 30 minutes

29) *If urine is refrigerated, how long can it be kept for?*
   a) Up to 24 hours
   b) Up to 6 hours
   c) Up to 2 hours
   d) Up to 30 minutes

30) *The specific gravity range for dog urine is:*
   a) 1:010–1:050
   b) 1:020–1:040
   c) 1:018–1:045
   d) 1:025–1:065

31) *The specific gravity range for cat urine is:*
   a) 1:010–1:050
   b) 1:020–1:040
   c) 1:018–1:045
   d) 1:025–1:065

32) *An increased specific gravity may be due to:*
   a) polydipsia
   b) Diabetes Insipidus
   c) pyometra
   d) dehydration

33) *Which ONE of the following crystals is found in alkaline urine?*

   a) Urates
   b) Oxalates
   c) Cystine
   d) Phosphates

34) *Which ONE of the following crystals is often found in Dalmatians' urine?*

   a) Urates
   b) Oxalates
   c) Cystine
   d) Phosphates

35) *In which type of poisoning may calcium oxalate crystals occur?*

   a) Warfarin
   b) Ethylene glycol
   c) Metaldehyde
   d) Paraquat

36) *Uroliths are:*

   a) stones formed within a body cavity
   b) stones formed from urine crystals
   c) stones formed from cells
   d) stones formed from casts

37) *Bacteria called cocci are:*

   a) rod-shaped
   b) spiral in shape
   c) square in shape
   d) round in shape

38) *Bacteria called bacilli are:*

   a) rod-shaped
   b) spiral in shape
   c) square in shape
   d) round in shape

39) *To examine the morphology of bacteria, which stain should be used?*

   a) Leishman's stain
   b) Methylene blue stain
   c) Gram stain
   d) Sudan III

40) *A cultural medium used to grow ringworm is:*

   a) nutrient agar
   b) McConkey agar
   c) chocolate agar
   d) Sabouraud's agar

41) *The mordant in a Gram stain is the:*

   a) distilled water
   b) acetone
   c) Lugol's iodine
   d) crystal violet

42) *Gram negative bacteria stain:*

   a) blue
   b) green
   c) orange
   d) red

43) *Gram positive bacteria stain:*

   a) blue
   b) green
   c) orange
   d) red

44) *The stain used to detect acid fast bacteria is:*

   a) methylene blue
   b) Ziehl-Neelsen stain
   c) Gram stain
   d) Leishman's stain

45) *What colour do non acid fast organisms stain?*

   a) Red
   b) Blue
   c) Orange
   d) Green

46) *At what temperature should inoculated bacteriology plates be incubated?*

   a) 34°C
   b) 36°C
   c) 37°C
   d) 40°C

47) *Which medium is used for growing salmonellae?*

   a) Blood agar
   b) Chocolate agar
   c) McConkey agar
   d) Deoxycholate citrate agar

48) *How long should inoculated plates be left in the incubator for?*

   a) 6–12 hours
   b) 12–24 hours
   c) 24–36 hours
   d) 48 hours or more

49) *Haemobartonella felis is thought to be carried by fleas; which term BEST describes the way the fleas act as carriers?*

   a) As biological vectors
   b) As intermediate hosts
   c) As transport hosts
   d) As paratenic hosts

50) *What is a saprophyte?*

   a) An organism that lives on a larger organism and causes disease
   b) An organism that lives on dead or decaying organic matter
   c) An organism that benefits its host
   d) An organism that causes no harm nor good to its host

51) *Viral diseases can be positively diagnosed in the live animal using which of the following methods?*

   a) histology
   b) clinical signs
   c) rising antibody titre
   d) a single measurement of serum antibody levels

52) *For barrier nursing, all of the following statements are true EXCEPT:*

   a) nurses should wear waterproof aprons, gloves and boots
   b) they should treat isolated patients before the remainder of the inpatients
   c) animals in isolation should have their own sets of food bowls, cleaning utensils, grooming equipment and bedding
   d) animals with the same disease can be placed together in an isolation ward

53) *Which ONE of the following is a suitable disinfectant for cleaning a parvovirus contaminated area?*

   a) cetrimide
   b) chlorhexidine
   c) hypochlorite
   d) pine oil disinfectant

54) *Cerebellar hypoplasia in kittens may be caused by infection while in utero by:*

   a) FeLV
   b) FCA
   c) FIA
   d) FIE

55) *For which ONE of the following organisms that cause respiratory disease is no vaccine currently available?*

a) Bordetella bronchoseptica
b) Canine adenovirus
c) Canine herpes virus
d) Canine parainfluenza virus

56) *The drug group of choice in the treatment of feline pneumonitis and feline infectious anaemia is:*

a) the cephalosporins
b) the penicillins
c) the tetracyclines
d) tyloson

57) *Which ONE of the following ectoparasites commonly acts as a vector for a viral disease?*

a) Cheyletiella
b) Demodex canis
c) Sarcoptes scabiei
d) Spilopsyllus cuniculi

58) *Which ONE of the following is an example of an adjuvant?*

a) Aluminium hydroxide
b) Ferrous sulphate
c) Sodium chloride
d) Sterile water

59) *In what year was the Health and Safety At Work Act introduced?*

   a) 1965
   b) 1974
   c) 1985
   d) 1995

60) *For how long do accident books have to be kept?*

   a) 2 years
   b) 3 years
   c) 4 years
   d) 5 years

61) *Which part of the microscope allows us to record a reference for re-location of an object on a slide?*

   a) The axis
   b) The mechanical stage
   c) The objective stage
   d) The vernier scale

62) *When posting an individual pathological sample, the size of the container must NOT exceed:*

   a) 100 ml
   b) 75 ml
   c) 50 ml
   d) 25 ml

63) *When preserving tissue samples for toxicology, the best preservative is:*

   a) 10% normal saline
   b) toluene
   c) boric acid
   d) 95% ethanol

64) *Containers for dispatch of tissue samples SHOULD be:*

   a) narrow-necked
   b) wide-necked
   c) snap-on top
   d) made of aluminium

65) *Synovial fluid is collected via:*

   a) pericardiocentesis
   b) thoracocentesis
   c) paracentesis
   d) arthrocentesis

66) *For which ONE of the following is AUTOLYSIS the best description?*

   a) Digestion of tissue by its own enzymes
   b) Destruction of red blood cells
   c) Destruction of white blood cells
   d) Digestion of platelets

67) *Which ONE of the following is NOT considered to be zoonotic?*

a) Ixodes
b) Notoedres
c) Demodex
d) Ctenocephalides

68) *How SHOULD used culture plates be disposed of?*

a) Put into a clinical waste bag
b) Disinfected and put in a clinical waste bag
c) Autoclaved and put in a black bag
d) Autoclaved and put in a clinical waste bag

69) *What is a microhaematocrit centrifuge used for?*

a) To obtain a serum sample
b) To measure packed cell volume
c) To obtain deposit from a urine sample
d) To perform a worm egg count

70) *What is the thoma pipette used for?*

a) Urinalysis
b) Bacteriology
c) Red blood cell and white blood cell counts
d) As a dropping pipette

71) *What is the function of the vernier scale?*

   a) Controls the amount of light
   b) Adjusts the eyepieces
   c) Relocates the object
   d) Moves the slide

72) *What does a DECREASE in PCV indicate?*

   a) Anaemia
   b) Dehydration
   c) Leucopenia
   d) Increase in basophils

73) *What is Leishman's stain used for?*

   a) To identify gram + ve bacteria
   b) To stain a blood smear for identifying white blood cells
   c) To stain haemoparasites
   d) To identify the shape of bacteria

74) *Which ONE of the following may cause a neutrophilia?*

   a) Bone marrow suppression
   b) Allergy
   c) Leukaemia
   d) Acute blood infection

75) *What is boric acid used for?*

  a) As a urine preservative
  b) An anticoagulant
  c) As a preservative for tumours
  d) As a purgative

76) *Are triple phosphate crystals most commonly formed in:*

  a) alkaline urine
  b) acid urine
  c) neutral urine
  d) acid or alkaline urine

77) *How would you microscopically identify starch granules in a faecal sample?*

  a) As striations
  b) As clear bubbles
  c) As black dots
  d) As red dots

78) *What is the first stain used in a Gram stain?*

  a) Methylene blue
  b) Grams iodine
  c) Giemsa stain
  d) Crystal violet stain

79) *What type of urine crystals are MOST commonly found in cats?*

 a) Calcium oxalate crystals
 b) Uric acid crystals
 c) Struvite crystals
 d) Cystine crystals

80) *What is the normal packed cell volume (PCV) range of the dog?*

 a) 25–45%
 b) 37–55%
 c) 40–58%
 d) 45–62%

81) *Which ONE of the following is NOT a Zoonoses?*

 a) Ctenocephalides canis
 b) Otodectes cyanotis
 c) Cheyletiella Spp
 d) Sarcoptes Scabiei

82) *Which colour container does the anti-coagulant EDTA usually come in?*

 a) Green
 b) Grey
 c) Yellow
 d) Pink

83) *Which ONE of the following worm eggs are identified under a microscope as being lemon-shaped, with a thick wall and polar caps?*

   a) Toxocara canis
   b) Dipylidium caninum
   c) Coccidia
   d) Trichuris vulpis

84) *Looking at a faeces sample under the microscope, what shows up as black dots?*

   a) Muscle fibres
   b) Fat globules
   c) Starch granules
   d) Worm eggs

85) *A refractometer measures urine:*

   a) pH
   b) protein
   c) blood
   d) specific gravity

86) *Which ONE of the following is a cestode?*

   a) Toxocara canis
   b) Toxocara leonina
   c) Dipylidum caninum
   d) Trichuris vulpis

87) *Which ONE of the following preserves urine without interfering with bacteriology and routine urinalysis?*

   a) Formalin
   b) Toluene
   c) Thymol
   d) Boric acid

88) *Which parasite has eight legs, is oval in shape and has trumpets on the end of its legs?*

   a) Otodectes
   b) Cheyletiella
   c) Sarcoptes
   d) Trichodectes

89) *Which ONE of the following parasites is a vector for Lyme disease?*

   a) Ctenocephelides felis
   b) Trombicula autumnalis
   c) Notoedres cati
   d) Ixodes

90) *Catheterization is essential if a urine sample is to be examined for:*

   a) protein
   b) bacteria
   c) blood
   d) glucose

91) *A spectrophotometer is used to:*
   a) measure enzyme levels in the blood
   b) measure glucose levels in the blood
   c) perform a red blood cell count
   d) culture ringworm

92) *Disintegration caused by blood being stored at too high a temperature is called:*
   a) desiccation
   b) haemolysis
   c) autolysis
   d) coagulation

93) *When preserving pathological specimens, the volume of formalin SHOULD:*
   a) exceed 10 times formalin to tissue
   b) exceed 20 times formalin to tissue
   c) exceed 3 times formalin to tissue
   d) exceed 5 times formalin to tissue

94) *Which ONE of the following preservatives is particularly toxic to humans?*
   a) Boric acid
   b) Acid citrate dextrose
   c) Normal saline
   d) Toluene

95) *Serological examination of the blood is of:*

   a) the appearance, size and numbers of blood cells in the blood
   b) poisons in the blood
   c) levels of antibodies in the blood
   d) the presence of Haemobartonella felis in the blood

96) *Which ONE of the following methods is NOT used to diagnose ringworm?*

   a) Skin scrape
   b) Coat brushing
   c) Wood's lamp
   d) Culture

97) *What is an antihelminthic?*

   a) A drug used to neutralise the activity of gastric juice
   b) A drug which prevents blood clotting
   c) A drug which neutralises the effect of histamines
   d) A drug which expels or destroys internal parasites

98) *Which ONE of the following is not a nematode?*

   a) Uncinaria stenocephala
   b) Dipylidium caninum
   c) Oclerus osleri
   d) Toxocara canis

99) *Name TWO cestodes found in the dog and cat:*

    a) Dipylidium caninum and Trichuris vulpis

    b) Dipylidium caninum and Taenia taeniaeformis

    c) Trichuris vulpis and Toxocara canis

    d) Uncinaria stenocephala and Taenia taeniaeformis

100) *What animal is Trichuris vulpis MOST likely to be found in?*

    a) pet rabbits

    b) kennelled dogs

    c) domesticated cats

    d) farm animals

101) *The formation of renal calculi may be enhanced by:*

    a) antibiotics

    b) cytotoxic drugs

    c) diuretic drugs

    d) corticosteroids

102) *What are rouleaux?*

    a) A stain used to detect blood parasites

    b) Grouping of red blood cells in stacks

    c) Nuclear remnants in a cell

    d) Red blood cells showing irregular margins and prickly edges

103) *Which reagents are necessary for performing a Gram stain?*

   a) Carbol fuschin, acid alcohol, methylene blue
   b) Carbol fuschin, Lugol's iodine, methylene blue and acetone
   c) Crystal violet, Lugol's iodine, acetone and saffranine
   d) Crystal violet, methylene blue, acetone and saffranine

104) *What does ELISA stand for?*

   a) Enzyme-leukaemia immunosorbent assay
   b) Enzyme-leukaemia assay
   c) Enzyme-linked immune assay
   d) Enzyme-linked immunosorbent assay

105) *Into which anticoagulant would you collect dog or cat blood for routine haematological examination?*

   a) EDTA
   b) Heparin
   c) Sodium citrate
   d) Sodium fluoride

106) *Leishman's stain is commonly used for:*

   a) bacterial staining
   b) differential white cell count
   c) total red cell count
   d) urinalysis

107) *Polycythemia is:*

    a) an increase in the number of blood platelets
    b) an increase in the number of red blood cells
    c) an increase in the number of white blood cells
    d) variable size of red blood cells

108) *How long can a serum sample be stored in a refrigerator without deterioration?*

    a) A few hours only
    b) 3 days
    c) 7 days
    d) 28 days

109) *What type of light is produced by a Wood's lamp?*

    a) Infrared
    b) Infrared and ultraviolet
    c) Ultraviolet
    d) Ultraviolet and visible light

110) *Sudan III is used in the laboratory to estimate the quantity of which ONE of the following?*

    a) Faecal fat
    b) Protein in urine
    c) Reticulocytes in peripheral blood
    d) Serum bicarbonate

111) *Which ONE of the following parasites can NOT be diagnosed by a skin scraping or brushing?*

   a) Cheyletiella
   b) Dipylidium caninum
   c) Helminth dermatoses
   d) Sarcoptes scabiei

112) *A laboratory test shows an increase in serum protein. Which ONE of the following is a possible cause?*

   a) Anaemia
   b) Dehydration
   c) Over hydration
   d) Renal failure

113) *Which ONE of the following media would NOT be used for growing Salmonella?*

   a) Nutrient agar
   b) Deoxycholate citrate
   c) MacConkey's agar
   d) Selenite broth

114) *Which ONE of the following parasites is found living within hair follicles?*

   a) Cnemidocoptes
   b) Demodex
   c) Notoedres
   d) Sarcoptes

115) *Which ONE of the following statements is NOT true?*

   a) Adult ticks have four pairs of legs
   b) All mites that affect cats are permanent parasites
   c) Juvenile ticks have only three pairs of legs
   d) Only the immature form of Trombicula autumnalis is parasitic

116) *Which ONE of the following may cause haemolysis in a blood sample?*

   a) Leaving the plasma unseparated in transit
   b) The use of too fine a needle to collect the sample
   c) Water on the needle or syringe
   d) All of the above

117) *Which ONE of the following statements is NOT true?*

   a) A lymphopaenia may be found in chemotherapy patients
   b) Eosinophilia is often found in cases of parasitism
   c) Neutropenia is usually seen in infectious inflammatory conditions
   d) Thrombocytopaenia may result in haemorrhage

118) *The flea species found MOST commonly on pet dogs is:*

   a) Cnemidocoptes
   b) Ctenocephalides canis
   c) Ctenocephalides felis
   d) Pulex irritans

119) *Which ONE of the following statements is the MOST accurate?*

   a) Dipylidium caninum may affect humans
   b) Dipylidium caninum may affect the cat as well as the dog
   c) The louse may be an intermediate host of Dipylidium caninum
   d) All of the above

120) *Dipylidium caninum infestation causes disease in the final host by:*

   a) competition for nutrients with the host
   b) causing diarrhoea
   c) loss of blood from the intestinal wall
   d) Dipylidium caninum rarely causes overt disease in the final host

121) *Which ONE of the following statements concerning Echinococcus granulosus is NOT true?*

   a) Even a few worms in the final host can cause severe diarrhoea
   b) Only one of the two subspecies of E.granulosus is thought to be zoonotic
   c) The adult worm is about 0.5 cm long
   d) Within Great Britain, hydatid disease is most common in Wales

122) *The active ingredient in Panacur is:*

   a) Fenbendazole
   b) Mebendazole
   c) Nitroscanate
   d) Oxfendazole

123) *Pups may have adult worms of Toxocara canis within their intestines by the time they are how old?*

   a) 10 days
   b) 2 weeks
   c) 5 weeks
   d) 8 weeks

124) *Which ONE of the following statements about Toxocara canis is NOT true?*

   a) After about 8 weeks of age, most of the ingested larvae pass directly from the intestine to muscle where they encyst
   b) In ideal conditions, a fertile Toxocara canis egg may develop to the infective stage in less than a week
   c) Puppies begin to develop immunity to Toxocara canis from about 7 weeks of age
   d) Toxocara eggs remain viable within the environment for up to 2 years

125) *Which ONE of the following are sensible precautions for a pregnant woman to take to avoid infection with Toxoplasma gondii?*

   a) Avoid eating sheep cheeses
   b) Have the family cat's blood tested for toxoplasmosis
   c) Wear rubber gloves when gardening
   d) All of the above

126) *What is the normal range for packed cell volume in the cat?*

   a) 25–45%
   b) 37–55%
   c) 40–58%
   d) 45–62%

127) *The most numerous blood cells in the circulation are:*

   a) basophils
   b) eosinophils
   c) erythrocytes
   d) lymphocytes

128) *Which blood cell has phagocytosis as its main function?*

   a) Eosinophil
   b) Erythrocte
   c) Monocyte
   d) Lymphocyte

129) *The destruction of erythrocytes is called:*

   a) anaemia
   b) haemophilia
   c) haemolysis
   d) erythropoiesis

130) *Which ONE of the following is not a route of transmission for human toxoplasmosis?*

   a) Cutaneous penetration
   b) Ingestion of tissue cysts in raw or uncooked meat
   c) Infected water (with oocysts)
   d) Nonpasteurised milk

131) *Lungworm is the common name of:*

   a) Aelurostrongylus abstrusus
   b) Dipylidium caninum
   c) Toxocara cati
   d) Toxocaris leonina

132) *Trichuris vulpis is a:*

   a) Bladder worm
   b) Lungworm
   c) Tracheal worm
   d) Whipworm

133) *Old blood in faeces is described as:*

    a) pathogenic
    b) melaena
    c) occult blood
    d) tenesmus

134) *When examined using UV light Microsporum canis usually fluoresces:*

    a) blue-green
    b) apple green
    c) yellow
    d) yellow-red

135) *Systemic ringworm infections are MOST commonly treated with:*

    a) chlorhexidine
    b) iodine tablets
    c) griseofulvin
    d) thiabendazole

136) *E coli is:*

    a) a Gram negative coccus
    b) a Gram negative bacillus
    c) a Gram positive coccus
    d) a Gram positive bacillus

137) *The field lens on a microscope is the:*

a) upper lens in the eye piece
b) lower lens in the eye piece
c) oil immersion lens
d) upper lens in the substage condenser

138) *A dog is presented at surgery with alopecia around the eyes and muzzle, without obvious pruritus. Which mite do you suspect?*

a) Otodectes cyanotis
b) Demodex canis
c) Sarcoptes scabiei
d) Cheyletiella yasguri

139) *The parasite which typically causes intense pruritus and crusting of the ear tips is:*

a) Demodex canis
b) Trichodectes canis
c) Cheyletiella yasguri
d) Sarcoptes scabiei

140) *The eggs of which parasite are glued to the hair shafts of its host?*

a) Ctenocephalides felis
b) Sarcoptes scabiei
c) Otodectes cyanotis
d) Linognathus setosus

141) *Trichodectes canis* has:

   a) four pairs of legs, a broad head and biting mouth parts
   b) four pairs of legs, a conical head and biting mouth parts
   c) three pairs of legs, a broad head and biting mouth parts
   d) three pairs of legs, a conical head and sucking mouth parts

142) *The specific gravity of a urine sample reads above the scale on the refractometer (greater than 1.035). You dilute the urine 1:2 with distilled water. The sample now reads 1.013. The recorded specific gravity will be:*

   a) 1.026
   b) 1.039
   c) 2.026
   d) 3.039

143) *Which regulation is there responsibility to report absences from work of three or more days involving an incident at work?*

   a) COSHH
   b) Fire precaution
   c) PPE
   d) RIDDOR

144) *Fluoride oxalate is an anti-coagulant. In which procedure should it be used?*

   a) Bile acid determination
   b) Determination of levels of clotting factors
   c) Glucose determination
   d) Platelet counts

145) *The fluid fraction obtained after clotted blood is centrifuged is:*

   a) interstitial fluid
   b) intracellular fluid
   c) plasma
   d) serum

146) *Which ONE of the following urinary crystals has a flat, regular hexagonal shape?*

   a) Ammonium urate
   b) Calcium oxalate
   c) Cystine
   d) Triple phosphate

147) *NORMAL cerebrospinal fluid is:*

   a) clear
   b) cloudy
   c) pink-tinged
   d) straw coloured

148) *Which ONE of the following worms is a public health risk because it causes hydatid cysts?*

   a) Dipylidium caninum
   b) Echinococcus granulosus
   c) Filaroides osleri
   d) Toxocara canis

149) *When Sudan III is applied to a faecal smear it stains:*

   a) starch granules orange
   b) fat droplets pink
   c) fat droplets orange
   d) muscle fibres pink

150) *The mordant in Gram stain is:*

   a) iodine
   b) methylene blue
   c) carbol fuchsin
   d) safranine

151) *The primary stain in Gram stain is:*

   a) iodine
   b) crystal violet
   c) safranine
   d) giemsa

152) *A Gram positive bacterium stained with methylene blue will stain:*

 a) purple
 b) red
 c) blue
 d) orange

153) *The commonest cause of dermatophytosis in the cat is:*

 a) Microsporum gypseum
 b) Candida albicans
 c) Microsporum canis
 d) Trichophyton mentagrophytes

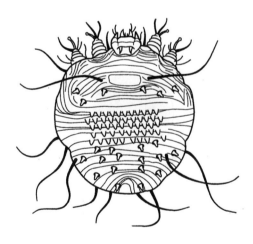

154) *The parasite in the diagram above is:*

 a) Demodex
 b) Sarcoptes
 c) Ctenocephalides felis
 d) Otodectes

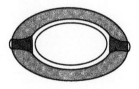

155) *The worm egg in the diagram above is:*

   a) Trichuris vulpis
   b) Toxocara cati
   c) Toxocaris leonina
   d) Taenia sp

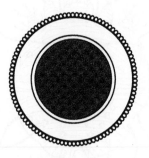

156) *The worm egg in the diagram above is:*

   a) Trichuris vulpis
   b) Toxocara canis
   c) Toxocaris leonina
   d) Taenia sp

157) *Which ONE of the following organisms is multicellular?*

   a) A bacterium
   b) A virus
   c) A fungus
   d) A protozoon

158) *The system used for naming micro-organisms is the:*

   a) binary system
   b) binomal system
   c) generic system
   d) Gram's system

159) *The term used to describe the genus to which micro-organisms belong is the:*

   a) generic name
   b) genetic name
   c) specific name
   d) species name

160) *Which ONE of the following bottles would NOT be used as a sample bottle?*

   a) McCartney bottle
   b) Universal container
   c) Erlenmyer flask
   d) Clean jam jar

161) *Which ONE of the following solutions is NOT used in Ziehl-Neelsen acid fast stain?*

   a) Carbol fuchsin
   b) Acid alcohol
   c) Lugol's iodine
   d) Methylene blue

162) *Fleas MAY be involved in the transmission of:*

   a) myxomatosis
   b) parvovirus
   c) FIA
   d) A & C

163) *Treatment for fleas on the host includes:*

   a) luferon
   b) permethrin
   c) negasunt
   d) fenbendazole

164) *Which ONE of the following is the biting louse of the dog?*

   a) Linognathus setosus
   b) Felicola subrostratus
   c) Trichodectes canis
   d) Ixodes ricinus

165) *Trichodectes canis is the intermediate host for:*

a) Ixodes ricinus
b) Panleucopaenia
c) Dipylidium caninum
d) Felicola subrostratus

166) *Ixodes hexagonus is the:*

a) sheep tick
b) hedgehog flea
c) hedgehog tick
d) sheep flea

167) *Which ONE of the following is described as a subsurface mite?*

a) Sarcoptes scabiei
b) Otodectes cyanotis
c) Cheyletilla yasguri
d) Trichodetes canis

168) *Cestode parasites are commonly known as:*

a) roundworms
b) hookworms
c) tapeworms
d) whipworms

169) *Which ONE of the following types of endoparasite is characteristically hermaphrodite?*

   a) Roundworm
   b) Hookworm
   c) Tapeworm
   d) Whipworm

170) *The correct term for the head of a cestode parasite is:*

   a) the rostellum
   b) the scolex
   c) the proscolex
   d) the proglottid

171) *The term for a mature tapeworm segment which contains fertilised eggs is:*

   a) granulid
   b) glenoid
   c) gravid
   d) none of the above

172) *The cell wall of a bacterium is comprised of:*

   a) peptidoglycan
   b) peptidases
   c) polypeptides
   d) pepsin

173) *The Health and Safety at Work Act (1974) applies to:*
    a) The practice principal
    b) The veterinary surgeons
    c) The veterinary nurses
    d) everyone

174) *Conjugation is a means by which genetic material is passed from one bacterium to another. The extra genetic material transmitted is called:*
    a) a pilus
    b) a plasmid
    c) plasma
    d) a recipient

175) *Blood agar can be used for culturing bacteria under laboratory conditions. How much animal blood does the blood agar contain?*
    a) 1%
    b) 10%
    c) 20%
    d) 50%

176) *Blood cells showing irregular margins and prickly points are known as:*
    a) crenated
    b) rouleaux
    c) proerythroblasts
    d) icteric

177) *Agar is commonly used in culture media for bacterial cultivation. It is made from:*

   a) extract of seaweed
   b) gelatin
   c) starch
   d) gelatinous mass

178) *Which ONE of the following terms is used to describe a bacterium that can synthesise its own food?*

   a) heterotroph
   b) autotroph
   c) saprophyte
   d) parasite

179) *Which ONE of the following parasites could be described as mutualistic?*

   a) Toxocara canis
   b) Ruminal gut micro-organisms
   c) Escherichia coli
   d) Toxocara cati

180) *A bacterium that is a facultative anaerobe is one that:*

   a) requires a good supply of oxygen
   b) requires a good supply of carbon dioxide
   c) grows best when oxygen concentration is lower than atmospheric air
   d) grows when oxygen is present but only functions in the absence of oxygen

181) *In choosing antibiotics, what is meant by potentiation?*

    a) The antibiotic is effective against Gram negative bacteria

    b) The antibiotic is effective against a range of bacteria

    c) Two antibiotics work together to enhance each other's effectiveness

    d) One antibiotic interacts undesirably with another

182) *Which urinary cast is clear, cylindrical, colourless and refractile and will dissolve in alkaline urine?*

    a) Tubular

    b) Hyaline

    c) Cellular

    d) Waxy

183) *Bacteria exist in a variety of shapes. How would you classify these bacteria?*

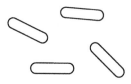

    a) Bacilli

    b) Vibrii

    c) Cocci

    d) Spirochaetes

184) *Which ONE of the following agar media would be most suitable for the culture of bacteria from a faecal sample?*

   a) blood agar
   b) chocolate agar
   c) MacConkey agar
   d) Deoxycholate citrate agar

185) *Plasma samples can be stored in the fridge for up to:*

   a) 24 hours
   b) 3 days
   c) 1 week
   d) 3 weeks

186) *Raised total protein levels in a blood sample may be due to:*

   a) dehydration
   b) debility
   c) decreased protein synthesis
   d) pathological loss of protein

187) *Hypernatremia is:*

   a) increased blood sodium concentration
   b) increased blood calcium concentration
   c) increased blood potassium concentration
   d) increased blood phosphorus concentration

188) *Hyperkalemia is:*

   a) increased blood sodium concentration
   b) increased blood calcium concentration
   c) increased blood potassium concentration
   d) increased blood phosphorus concentration

189) *Normal range of plasma urea concentration in the dog is:*

   a) 0–22 mmoll
   b) 2–8 mmoll
   c) 8–16 mmoll
   d) 16–24 mmoll

190) *High plasma urea may be seen in cases of:*

   a) renal failure
   b) diabetes mellitus
   c) Cushing's disease
   d) hyperthyroidism

191) *Creatinine levels are most commonly used in diagnostic aids to indicate:*

   a) renal conditions
   b) thyroid conditions
   c) liver conditions
   d) cardiovascular conditions

192) *The eggs of Toxocara canis appear in faeces as*

    a) darkly nucleated, with a pitted shell
    b) darkly nucleated, with a smooth shell
    c) with a pale nucleus and a pitted shell
    d) with a pale nucleus and a smooth shell

193) *The segment of a tapeworm is described as a*

    a) strobilla
    b) gravid
    c) proglottid
    d) rostellum

194) *Which ONE of these animal species would it be appropriate to starve prior to sampling?*

    a) Bovine
    b) Canine
    c) Feline
    d) Lapine

195) *Under which of the following pieces of legislation is it necessary to report serious injuries that occur in the practice laboratory?*

    a) COSHH 99
    b) RIDDOR 95
    c) HSAWA 74
    d) Environmental protection Act 1990

196) *Which ONE of the following parts of the microscope is responsible for regulating light?*

    a) Eye piece
    b) Objective lens
    c) Course adjustment
    d) Iris diaphragm

197) *The nose piece of the light microscope contains:*

    a) the objective lenses
    b) the eyepieces
    c) the sub stage condenser
    d) the course adjustment

198) *Bacteria should be viewed first on which ONE of the following magnifications:*

    a) $\times 4$
    b) $\times 10$
    c) $\times 40$
    d) $\times 100$

199) *Felicola subrostratus should be examined under which of the following objectives?*

    a) $\times 4$
    b) $\times 10$
    c) $\times 40$
    d) $\times 100$

200) *Which ONE of the following fluids contains clotting factors?*

   a) Serum
   b) Plasma
   c) Interstitial fluid
   d) Intracellular fluid

201) *The function of a Diff-Quick stain is to:*

   a) stain a smear for haematological examination
   b) stain a smear for bacteriological examination
   c) stain a smear for urine examination
   d) stain a smear for faecal examination

202) *What colour is the container for a blood sample that is to be placed in sodium fluoride?*

   a) Orange
   b) Pink
   c) Yellow
   d) Uncoloured

203) *Which ONE of the following blood cell types is seen LEAST commonly in the normal blood smear of the dog?*

   a) Basophil
   b) Neutrophil
   c) Eosinophil
   d) Lymphocyte

204) *Which ONE of the following white blood cells is agranular?*

a) Neutrophil
b) Eosinophil
c) Basophil
d) Monocyte

205) *The Unopette method may be used in which ONE of the following types of examinations?*

a) Haemotological
b) Biochemical
c) Bacteriological
d) Faecal

206) *The PCV of a cat may increase in which ONE of the following situations*

a) Anaemia
b) Overhydration
c) Dehydration
d) Haemobartenella infection

207) *Which ONE of the following parasites has eight legs?*

a) Flea
b) Tick
c) Biting louse
d) Sucking louse

208) *Geimsa stain may be used in which ONE of the following types of investigation?*

   a) Haematology
   b) Urinalysis
   c) Bacteriology
   d) Biochemistry

209) *The fluid used for total white blood cell estimation is known as:*

   a) Turk's solution
   b) saline
   c) Lugol's Iodine
   d) crystal Violet

210) *Which ONE of the following would improve contrast when using a light microscope?*

   a) Iris diaphram
   b) Substage condenser
   c) Huyghen lenses
   d) Immersion oil

211) *Ethylenediamine tetra-acetic acid (EDTA) is the anticoagulant of choice for haematology because it:*

   a) preserves blood cell morphology
   b) simultaneously stains and preserves blood cells
   c) destroys red cells while preserving white cells
   d) destroys white cells while preserving red cells

212) *Which lens is responsible for focusing light?*

   a) Huyghen
   b) Substage condenser
   c) Iris
   d) × 10 objective

213) *Most anticoagulants work by:*

   a) removing calcium from the plasma
   b) chelating potassium
   c) forming insoluble complexes with sodium
   d) removing fibrinogen

214) *Which anticoagulant inhibits a glycotic enzyme, thus acting as a preservative for glucose?*

   a) Sodium citrate
   b) Lithium heparin
   c) Sodium fluoride
   d) Potassium oxalate

215) *Serum should be separated from blood cells in a blood sample as soon as possible because:*

   a) it evaporates rapidly
   b) it will not clot
   c) it becomes lipaemic
   d) certain chemical constituents change if serum is allowed to stay in contact with cells

216) *All of the following may cause haemolysis except:*

   a) removing the needle from the syringe to place blood in a collection tube
   b) freezing a whole blood sample
   c) mixing too vigorously after sample collection
   d) forcing blood sample through the needle

217) *If you are unable to carry out biochemical tests on a sample for a few days, you should:*

   a) centrifuge the sample, separate the serum, and freeze it
   b) place the sample in the refrigerator
   c) centrifuge the sample and freeze it
   d) centrifuge the sample and refrigerate it

218) *Performing a group of blood chemistry tests to evaluate the overall health of an animal is referred to as:*

   a) biochemical profiling
   b) quality control assurance
   c) a complete blood count
   d) a differential diagnosis

219) *The anticoagulant used to preserve blood glucose levels for blood chemistry analysis is:*

   a) EDTA
   b) sodium or lithium heparin
   c) sodium or lithium oxalate
   d) sodium fluoride

220) *The preferred sample for most blood chemistry tests is:*
   a) whole blood
   b) serum
   c) plasma
   d) urine

221) *To preserve blood constituents in the event that sample analysis is delayed, serum or plasma should be:*
   a) lyophilized and reconstituted before analysis
   b) refrigerated and warmed to room temperature before analysis
   c) placed in a 37°C water bath and brought to room temperature before analysis
   d) placed at room temperature until analysed

222) *A blood sample from an animal that has recently eaten may be:*
   a) haemolysed
   b) lipaemic
   c) icteric
   d) anaemic

223) *Centrifuging a blood sample at high speed for a prolonged period may result in:*
   a) lipaemia
   b) icterus
   c) haemolysis
   d) bacterial contamination

224) *Improper handling of a blood sample, including vigorous shaking or forcing through a needle, may result in:*

 a) lipaemia
 b) icterus
 c) haemolysis
 d) bacterial contamination

225) *A serum sample that is extremely icteric generally derives its colour from an increased level of:*

 a) lipids
 b) total bilirubin
 c) electrolytes
 d) glucose

226) *A box of reagents for blood chemistry analysis labelled for storage at 8°C can be safely stored*

 a) in the freezer
 b) at room temperature
 c) in the incubator
 d) in the refrigerator

227) *The technology of dry chemistry differs from that of wet chemistry in that the reagents in dry chemistry are supplied:*

 a) in lyophilized pellets
 b) in liquid solutions
 c) impregnated on slides, cards, or strips
 d) in powdered capsules

228) *Which stain is used to confirm the presence of fat in a faecal smear?*

   a) New methylene blue
   b) Sudan III or IV
   c) Diff-Quick
   d) Giemsa

229) *Which stain is referred to as a supravital stain?*

   a) New methylene blue
   b) Camco-Quick
   c) Eosin
   d) Sudan III or IV

230) *Which ONE of the following pipettes is NOT graduated?*

   a) Marburg
   b) Thoma
   c) Serological
   d) Pasteur

231) *For what purpose are Unopettes used in haematology?*

   a) Blood cell count
   b) Hematocrit determination
   c) Haemoglobin determination
   d) Total protein determination

232) *What term describes a subnormal neutrophil count?*

   a) Leucocytosis
   b) Neutropaenia
   c) Anaemia
   d) Regenerate left shift

233) *Which cell becomes a macrophage once it enters the tissues?*

   a) Plasma cell
   b) Lymphocyte
   c) Neutrophil
   d) Monocyte

234) *Which ONE of the following is an intracellular parasite of erythrocytes?*

   a) Babesia
   b) Ehrlichia
   c) Trypanosoma
   d) Toxoplasma

235) *Granular casts in urine are associated with:*

   a) inflammatory change
   b) chronic degenerative renal tubular changes
   c) poor circulation
   d) normal urine

236) *What is the term used to describe plasma that appears white or milky?*

   a) leukaemia
   b) lipaemia
   c) leucocytosis
   d) icterus

237) *For how long must the typical microhaematocrit tube be centrifuged for packed cell volume determination?*

   a) 1 min
   b) 5 min
   c) 10 min
   d) 15 min

238) *Howell-Jolly bodies resemble which erythrocyte parasite?*

   a) Babesia
   b) Haemobartonella
   c) Trypanosoma
   d) Ehrlichia

239) *What is NORMALLY the largest blood cell in domestic species?*

   a) Monocyte
   b) Neutrophil
   c) Eosinophil
   d) Lymphocyte

240) *Which leucocyte can normally have a bean-shaped nucleus?*

   a) Lymphocyte
   b) Plasma cell
   c) Monocyte
   d) Band neutrophil

241) *An increased number of band cells in the peripheral blood indicates:*

   a) leukaemia
   b) autoimmune haemolytic anaemia
   c) a left shift
   d) neutropaenia

242) *Alanine aminotransferase (ALT) readings are sometimes used in the dog to indicate:*

   a) lymphatic damage
   b) cardiovascular damage
   c) renal damage
   d) hepatic damage

243) *The ACTH stimulation test is essential for the confirmation of:*

   a) Addison's disease
   b) diabetes mellitus
   c) Cushing's syndrome
   d) hyperthryoidism

244) *To examine microscopically the sediment from a urine sample, the sample should be spun for:*

    a) 5 min at 2000 rpm

    b) 4 min at 8000 rpm

    c) 3 min at 10,000 rpm

    d) 2 min at 6000 rpm

245) *The function of the Huyghen lens is to:*

    a) distinguish between black and white

    b) obtain good contrast

    c) focus light onto the object

    d) magnify the primary image

246) *Ketone bodies in a urine sample may indicate to the vet that the animal is suffering from:*

    a) Addison's disease

    b) Cushing's syndrome

    c) diabetes inspidus

    d) diabetes mellitus

247) *The total magnification of an object using ×10 eyepiece and ×40 objective will be:*

    a) × 10

    b) × 40

    c) × 50

    d) × 400

248) *Large numbers of hyaline casts may be present in a urine sample if the animal is suffering from:*

a) renal failure
b) diabetes mellitus
c) diabetes insipidus
d) Cushing's syndrome

249) *In acid urine, which ONE of the following crystals is MOST likely to be present?*

a) Uric acid
b) Triple phosphate
c) Carbonate
d) Ammonium magnesium phosphate

250) *For cellular examination, a sample of cerebrospinal fluid should be placed in a:*

a) plain tube
b) EDTA tube
c) heparin tube
d) oxalate tube

251) *Cerebrospinal fluid samples may clot in a plain blood tube due to their high:*

a) protein content
b) white blood cell content
c) red blood cell content
d) haemoglobin content

252) *Normal cerebrospinal fluid is:*

   a) yellow, turgid and odourless
   b) clear, turgid and odourless
   c) clear, transparent and odourless
   d) yellow, opaque and odourless

253) *The vein of choice to take a blood sample from a rabbit is the:*

   a) marginal ear vein
   b) cephalic vein
   c) saphenous vein
   d) jugular vein

254) *The vein of choice to take a blood sample from a young kitten is the:*

   a) marginal ear vein
   b) cephalic vein
   c) saphenous vein
   d) jugular vein

255) *For microhaematocrit readings, the capillary tube should be spun for:*

   a) 2 min at 10,000 rpm
   b) 5 min at 10,000 rpm
   c) 8 min at 4000 rpm
   d) 10 min at 2000 rpm

256) *The reticulocytes in the normal total red cell count in the cat and dog make up approximately:*

a) 1%
b) 10%
c) 15%
d) 20%

257) *The warning label with a skull and crossbones indicates that a chemical is:*

a) corrosive
b) harmful
c) highly inflammable
d) toxic

258) *The MOST commonly used stain for a differential white blood cell count is:*

a) methylene blue
b) Leishman's
c) Geimsa
d) Gram stain

259) *Haemobartonella felis is detected after staining a blood smear with:*

a) methylene blue
b) Leishman's
c) Geimsa
d) Gram stain

260) *Decreased lymphocyte numbers in a differential count may be due to:*
   a) dehydration
   b) shock
   c) lowered PCV
   d) lymphopaenia

261) *Eosinophils may be increased in the presence of:*
   a) diabetes inspidus
   b) low hydration status
   c) haemobartonella felis
   d) allergies or parasitism

262) *A reduced total white cell count is UNLIKELY to be due to:*
   a) bone marrow failure
   b) overwhelming infection
   c) viral disease
   d) allergic reaction

263) *Which ONE of the following is the MOST appropriate long-term preservative for mites:*
   a) surgical spirit
   b) mineral oil
   c) potassium hydroxide (KOH)
   d) DTX mountant

264) *Neotrombicula autumnali is also known as:*

   a) sarcoptes mange mite
   b) cat flea
   c) harvest mite
   d) walking dandruff

265) *Which ONE of the following solutions is NOT appropriate for the flotation of parasite eggs in a faeces examination?*

   a) Saturated salt solution
   b) Saturated sugar solution
   c) Saturated magnesium sulphate solution
   d) Saturated potassium hydroxide solution

266) *The McMasters slide is used for:*

   a) total red blood cell counts
   b) urine analysis
   c) faecal worm egg counts
   d) total protein estimation

267) *Confirmation of which ONE of the following parasites would require serological tests?*

   a) Toxoplasma gondii
   b) Toxocariasis
   c) Dipylidium caninim
   d) Haemobartonella felis

268) *Which ONE of the following is NOT an intestinal protozoon?*

   a) Toxoplasma
   b) Cryptosporidea
   c) Sarcocystis
   d) Taenia sp

269) *Which ONE of the following is NOT a respiratory tract nematode?*

   a) Oslerus osleri
   b) Filaroides hirthi
   c) Angiostrongylus vasorium
   d) Trichuris vulpis

270) *Which ONE of the following is NOT an intestinal nematode?*

   a) Echinococcus granulosus
   b) Uncinaria stenocephala
   c) Trichuris vulpis
   d) Toxocara canis

271) *Crenation of red blood cells results in:*

   a) shrinkage of the cells
   b) increased turgidity of the cells
   c) water moving in by osmosis
   d) water moving in by active transport

272) *Pyuria is:*

   a) pus in urine
   b) abnormal numbers of WBCs in circulation
   c) the presence of large numbers of WBCs in urine
   d) large numbers of red blood cells in the gut

273) *The suffix paenia refers to:*

   a) a decrease in the number of cells
   b) an increase in the number of cells
   c) a change in the number of cells
   d) fluctuating cell numbers

274) *The suffix philia refers to:*

   a) a decrease in the number of cells
   b) an increase in the number of cells
   c) a change in the number of cells
   d) fluctuating cell numbers

275) *Which ONE of the following media would be MOST appropriate for salmonella culture?*

   a) Sabourauds dextrose agar
   b) Deoxycholate citrate agar
   c) Blood agar
   d) Nutrient agar

276) *What is the function of a colorimeter?*

   a) It measures intensity of heat in a solution
   b) It measures intensity of colour in a solution
   c) It separates blood cells from plasma
   d) It separates faecal matter in a solution

277) *The smallest of the white blood cells is the:*

   a) lymphocyte
   b) neutrophil
   c) monocyte
   d) basophil

278) *Heparin is the anticoagulant of choice when:*

   a) plasma samples are required
   b) haematological examination is to take place
   c) glucose levels are under investigation
   d) serum samples are required

279) *In the dog, acute haemorrhage and icteric disease may be caused by:*

   a) bordetella bronchoseptica
   b) leptospira icterohaemorrhagiae
   c) parainfluenza
   d) parvovirus

280) *Blood agar is used for:*

   a) identification of ringworm spores
   b) routine isolation of aerobic bacteria
   c) isolation of enteric bacteria
   d) isolation of salmonella

281) *Staphylococci are:*

   a) rod-shaped and arranged in pairs
   b) spherical and arranged in pairs
   c) rod-shaped and arranged in clusters
   d) spherical and arranged in clusters

282) *Hair to be examined for dermatophyte investigation is best taken from:*

   a) the peripheral edges of the lesion
   b) the centre of the lesion
   c) anywhere within the lesion
   d) from outside the lesion

283) *The preferred method of urine sample collection for bacteriological investigation is:*

   a) mid stream voided sample collection
   b) catheterization
   c) bladder expression
   d) early morning sample collection

284) *The normal yellow colour of urine is due to the presence of:*

   a) proteins
   b) urochromes
   c) bile pigments
   d) haemoglobin

285) *In microscopy, magnification of an object is produced by:*

   a) the eyepiece
   b) the objective
   c) both the eyepiece and the objective
   d) the field lens

286) *Microscope slides to be used for blood smears should first be cleaned with:*

   a) detergent, and stored in ethanol
   b) surgical spirit
   c) soap, and stored in surgical spirit
   d) detergent, and stored in disinfectant

287) *For which ONE of the following microscopy examinations should oil immersion be used?*

   a) Identification of Demodex
   b) Identification of bacteria
   c) Identification of worm eggs
   d) Identification of urinary crystals

288) *A refractometer is used to measure:*

   a) urine glucose
   b) blood glucose
   c) urine specific gravity
   d) blood specific gravity

289) *The site of choice in the dog, for collection of blood for biochemical analysis is:*

   a) jugular vein
   b) saphenous vein
   c) sublingual artery
   d) carotid artery

290) *Plasma samples stored in the fridge can be kept for:*

   a) 24 hours
   b) 3 days
   c) 1 week
   d) 4 weeks

291) *Which ONE of the following is UNLIKELY to cause haemolysis in a collected sample:*

   a) inadequate mixing
   b) narrow gauge needle use
   c) wet needle use to collect blood
   d) forcing blood through the needle

292) *The following procedures all help to keep reagent strips in optimum condition, with the exception of:*

   a) storing away from high humidity
   b) not handling unnecessarily
   c) not returning unused strips to the container
   d) storing in the fridge

293) *Normal urine pH range for carnivores is:*

   a) 3–5
   b) 5–7
   c) 7–9
   d) 9–11

294) *Which ONE of the following is NOT a urinary calculus?*

   a) Cystine
   b) Urate
   c) Triple phosphate
   d) Hyaline cast

295) *Detection of haemobartonella felis is BEST undertaken using which ONE of the following stains?*

   a) Methylene blue
   b) Leishman's
   c) Giemsa
   d) Gram

296) *A shift to the left in haematological examination means:*

  a) increased immature neutrophils
  b) increased mature leucocytes
  c) decreased eosinophils
  d) decreased mature leucocytes

297) *A reduced white cell count is UNLIKELY to be due to:*

  a) bone marrow failure
  b) overwhelming infection
  c) viral disease
  d) allergic reaction

298) *Which ONE of the following parasitic infections is MOST likely to be diagnosed by collection of material from pustules:*

  a) Demodex
  b) Tryptophan
  c) Ctenocephalides
  d) Trichodectes

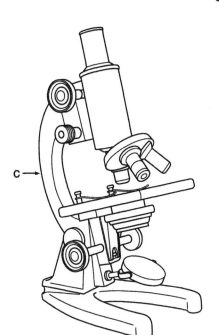

299) *In the picture above, identify the part labelled C as the:*

    a) substage condenser
    b) mechanical stage
    c) iris
    d) limb

300) *What size lenses are normally used in the microscope oculars?*

    a) × 6
    b) × 10
    c) × 40
    d) × 100

Answers

1)	a	23)	c	45)	a	67)	c
2)	c	24)	d	46)	c	68)	d
3)	b	25)	b	47)	d	69)	b
4)	d	26)	b	48)	b	70)	c
5)	c	27)	b	49)	c	71)	c
6)	a	28)	d	50)	b	72)	a
7)	d	29)	a	51)	c	73)	b
8)	d	30)	c	52)	b	74)	d
9)	a	31)	b	53)	c	75)	a
10)	c	32)	d	54)	d	76)	a
11)	c	33)	d	55)	c	77)	c
12)	a	34)	a	56)	c	78)	d
13)	c	35)	b	57)	d	79)	c
14)	b	36)	b	58)	a	80)	b
15)	d	37)	d	59)	b	81)	b
16)	c	38)	a	60)	a	82)	d
17)	b	39)	b	61)	d	83)	d
18)	b	40)	d	62)	c	84)	c
19)	c	41)	c	63)	d	85)	d
20)	b	42)	d	64)	b	86)	c
21)	d	43)	a	65)	d	87)	d
22)	c	44)	b	66)	a	88)	a

89)	d	125)	d	161)	c	197)	a
90)	b	126)	a	162)	d	198)	b
91)	a	127)	c	163)	b	199)	a
92)	a	128)	c	164)	c	200)	b
93)	a	129)	c	165)	c	201)	a
94)	d	130)	a	166)	c	202)	c
95)	c	131)	a	167)	a	203)	a
96)	b	132)	d	168)	c	204)	d
97)	d	133)	b	169)	a	205)	a
98)	b	134)	b	170)	b	206)	c
99)	b	135)	c	171)	c	207)	b
100)	b	136)	b	172)	a	208)	a
101)	c	137)	b	173)	d	209)	a
102)	b	138)	b	174)	b	210)	a
103)	c	139)	d	175)	b	211)	a
104)	d	140)	d	176)	a	212)	b
105)	a	141)	c	177)	a	213)	a
106)	b	142)	d	178)	b	214)	d
107)	b	143)	d	179)	b	215)	d
108)	a	144)	c	180)	c	216)	a
109)	c	145)	d	181)	c	217)	a
110)	a	146)	c	182)	b	218)	a
111)	b	147)	a	183)	a	219)	c
112)	b	148)	b	184)	d	220)	b
113)	a	149)	b	185)	b	221)	b
114)	b	150)	a	186)	a	222)	b
115)	d	151)	b	187)	a	223)	c
116)	d	152)	c	188)	c	224)	c
117)	c	153)	c	189)	b	225)	b
118)	c	154)	b	190)	a	226)	b
119)	d	155)	a	191)	a	227)	c
120)	d	156)	b	192)	a	228)	b
121)	a	157)	c	193)	c	229)	c
122)	a	158)	b	194)	b	230)	d
123)	b	159)	d	195)	b	231)	a
124)	a	160)	c	196)	d	232)	b

233)	d	250)	b	267)	a	284)	b
234)	a	251)	a	268)	d	285)	c
235)	a	252)	c	269)	d	286)	a
236)	b	253)	a	270)	a	287)	b
237)	b	254)	d	271)	a	288)	c
238)	b	255)	b	272)	c	289)	a
239)	a	256)	a	273)	a	290)	a
240)	c	257)	d	274)	b	291)	a
241)	c	258)	b	275)	b	292)	d
242)	d	259)	c	276)	b	293)	b
243)	c	260)	b	277)	a	294)	d
244)	a	261)	d	278)	a	295)	c
245)	d	262)	d	279)	b	296)	a
246)	d	263)	a	280)	b	297)	d
247)	d	264)	c	281)	d	298)	a
248)	a	265)	d	282)	a	299)	d
249)	a	266)	c	283)	b	300)	b

Printed and bound by CPI Group (UK) Ltd, Croydon, CR0 4YY

03/10/2024

01040848-0003